Do not give up your favorite sport because of a spine problem!

Preventive measures of spine disability.

Constantin Panow

COPYRIGHT 2013

The Holy Supper is kept, indeed, in whatso we share with another's need. Not what we give, but what we share, — For the gift without the giver is bare.

James Russell Lowell
American poet (1819-1891)

DISCLAIMER

The author and publisher decline responsibility about any injury or deleterious effect that could result from misinterpretation or wrong understanding and application of this text.

Consult with your physician before starting any training program!

KEY WORDS

Calisthenics, spinal disc herniation, scoliosis, spinal disability, prevention of scoliosis, prevention of disc herniation.

CONTENTS

PURPOSE OF TITLE

Nothing is more ominous to the modern human than having a spine problem.

As soon you tell somebody you have a disc herniation, people see you already in a rolling chair, or taking part in Paralympics.

Even specialists are reluctant to explaining to their patients too much about such a topic.

This is one of the reasons of this short text, aiming at better understanding in the public about problems of the spine.

It is not unusual to read in newspapers or a blog about a guy, who felt completely abandoned by professors in medicine.
They all foretold him he would never walk again; he is doomed in a roll chair forever.
That is what they mean most of the time, when they tell you that you are paraplegic.

That guy did not give up.
Not that he would not believe medical doctors.

Nothing similar!

He was just eager to exercise his body, as he had always done it.

And Miracle!

Two or three years later, not only he is exercising his arms and upper body like hell, but he is doing a few steps inside his flat.

He can move around for 10 to 20 meters (33 to 66 Feet) or so without help.

There is also the story of that other guy, using an exo-skeleton, developed by US Army for soldiers, supposed to carry some extra- luggage.

- Who is walking around like you and me, after he was left as paraplegic by specialists.

Those are fairy tales about true X-men of today!

No mutants!

Just guys who experiment with their bodies.

You could find certainly many similar stories, by no way fiction, apart from the fact that those guys found really something that worked for them.

Of course, rehabilitation surgeons and medical staff, they all know this topic better than me, and in case you need information, they would readily address you to the right community.

People who may help you with their advice recover not only your legs, but something more than that, confidence in your ability and your capacity to make your life in this world.

The topic of my book is a bit different.

ETIOLOGY OF SCOLIOSIS

In my practice I see rather what could have been done by public services and did not work.

There are more than 50 % people in this world who suffer from a slight scoliosis.

You would tell me: - What's the problem?
Anyway, your statistics is biased, because there was already a reason to do this X-Ray on these patients!
- How about prevention of scoliosis?
Of course, if you are an employee working in an office and doing some computer job, having a slight scoliosis would not hinder you from typewriting.
Everything changes if you are a heavy-duty worker of some kind, engaged for a construction firm or on a fuel platform on high sea...
Criteria for engagement are not even similar.
But many times, you start that job with eighteen and it is ok the first years.
I mean not only in the very first, but even during 10 or 20 years, you do this work without any inconvenience whatsoever.

And then, one day, you have a small accident.
Many times, it looks as if you just simply fell on a slippery surface.
Frequently a moment of inattention.
And from that day on, everything changes.
You go from doctor to a specialist.
They all tell you; they are going to deal with the problem, but the more it continues, the less you see yourself pursuing in the same job.
Many times, it is just a lumbar disc herniation.
Nothing special!
You have that operation, then re-education for a few weeks.
But when you try again to come back to work, you realize you just cannot do it anymore.
In the beginning it was just a slight scoliosis.

So, you would ask now: - How does a scoliosis evolve?
Of course, there are all these horrid cases of malformed children, some kind of syndrome, but this is rather the exception.
Most of the time, you were a completely normal child, and then something happened during growth!
Some cases are due to tethering of the cauda equine: - They call it spina bifida occulta.
Now we know it is often because your mom did not take any folic acid supplements when she was pregnant. This makes up for no more than 10 to 15 % of cases.

Most of the other ones develop scoliosis during maximal growth of skeleton.

We call it Scheuermann's disease.

What happens is that limiting plates of vertebrae lose their strength and just dissolve.

It is limited osteonecrosis of growth plates.

And you would ask me:

- How come?

For tens of years, we observed this phenomenon, and nobody knew what the cause was.

But since laboratories have the possibility to make dosage of vitamin D in blood:

- We know!

Most children living in temperate climates are deficient in vitamin D.

And some so badly, that they present with pain in many growing zones.

Bone can just not mature without this vitamin.

- And guess what?

- It becomes obvious, that not only Scheuermann's disease is due to such a deficit, but also what we were calling the osteochondroses.

- All these diseases described by different doctors almost one century ago.

- Like Seever's disease (calcaneal apophysitis)

- Osgood-Schlatter disease,

- And many more.

There were also those dense lines in metaphyses of long bones, which we would call curious names.

And when it was an adult, we would wonder whether he had had a heavy metal poisoning when he was a child, or some serious illness:

- All differentials that could be an explanation for this image.

- But most of the time, it was just Rickets, and nothing else.

And thus, USA sanitary authority rings alarm 2012, because a big percentage of the population in the Southern States is Vitamin D deficient!

What then about the Northern States?

One simple acknowledgement means, that many illnesses, crippling population of the Globe, are in fact preventable!

PREVENTION
OF SCOLIOSIS

It is sufficient to prescribe Vitamin D, as pills or solution!

At the same time a huge advertising takes place, which makes people hysterical about sunshine.
Because it gives skin cancer!
Sunbaths are supposed to give melanoma to every single person, who is enjoying them!
Unfortunately, advertising does not provide information about all diseases, which are induced in the absence of sufficient tanning of skin.
OK, scoliosis is one of them.
What experts do not tell you is that sunbaths strengthen your immunity.

And by doing so, prevent the appearance of many cancers of other organs, that would otherwise grow in your body.
And nobody tells you, that there is a right and a wrong way of taking a sunbath.
It is up to you to find out!
But, if you are reluctant to take some rays, and still

concerned for your health, you can prevent at least some of diseases that are bound to plague your health, by taking Vitamin D pills.

Do not forget your children, as it is even more important for a growing skeleton to have this essential element for one's development.

The medical community has not yet realized how tremendous this knowledge is, and how much adaptation it would need for a practitioner, to implement it in one's job.

As for instance, skeletal age in children.

A source still in use everywhere in the world is Radiographic Atlas of Skeletal Development of the Hand and Wrist, by William Greulich and S. Pyle, first published 1959.

Many of wrist X-Rays displayed in this excellent book harbor signs of rickets.

Well, you would say, it was half a century ago, and medical community did not know that children, who were considered normal, were in fact retarded by rickets.

And that children who were supposed retarded for unknown reasons.

- Well, we know today, that most of the time, it was because of deficit of Vitamin D.

Does this mean that all that Herculean work should be done again?

Well, what would be the normal children pool, on which we would do this work?

- As rickets is more prevalent than ever on the planet!

What this knowledge means, is that scoliosis is preventable in most cases:

- Simply by prescribing Vitamin D!
- Or summer vacations! (In the sun!)

And, so many other illnesses, that can have orthopedic implications sooner or later, are preventable by the same ways.

SCOLIOSIS IN THIRD AGE

Elderly people are frequently deficient in Vitamin B12.

Though abundant in our nutrition it needs the so-called intrinsic factor secreted by the stomach to be absorbed by the gut.

Because of auto-immune disease, parietal stomach cells decay in the elderly.

To prove this deficiency, dosing of this vitamin in blood plasma is not enough as levels remain in "normal" range.

Elevated Homocysteine levels are definite proof for this deficiency.

Methylmalonic levels can be also used.

PREVENTION OF SPINAL INJURY

But now we have a different problem also, to deal with:

- Boomers and their children have scoliosis to more than 50%.

What is to be done with this population, as deformed spine is no more correctable by modern means?

Nobody tells you, when you take a job, that you might get a problem with your back in a few years, because of scoliosis.

Is this also preventable?

As in any similar topic, the answer can be formulated only prudently.

If it concerns your sportive life, you will find it unjust, to limit it in any way, because of a minor flaw, would you?

But for a job, you should be overly critical!

- If you are supposed to carry heavy loads, then probably even people with slight scoliosis should be discouraged to engage.

But as in any matter! - You can always struggle to

improve odds!

If we try to materialize the Aim:

- How about preventing measures for disc herniation in slight scoliosis?

Sports community knows perfectly that you can condition every single part of your body.

- How about the vertebral spine?

CONDITIONING

Sports specialists propose you hundreds of exercises for every part of the body.

The only problem with this kind of thinking is that you do not know for what it is good.

And besides, you are so overwhelmed by the one hundred exercises, that you are supposed to do each day, that after a while, you simply give it all up.

- As every normal person! - You would say.

Medical doctors know that it is not only important to prescribe a treatment to an ill person.

- You must also make sure, that the patient would take it.

If it is too complicated, it is doomed to failure!

This is also the problem with modern Sports Industry.

- You absolutely need a boss to guide you in its complicated realm.

- And a personal trainer cost so much, that most people cannot afford for it.

Conditioning your vertebral spine needs some basic knowledge: - OK!

- But it is not SO complicated, that one cannot tell you the rules.

There are exercises, which should be avoided by all means:

- As for instance crunches!

Aerobics has probably no point in this topic, as it can be by itself deleterious to spinal health, in many of its forms.

- The answer is strength training.

Free weights are claimed to be safe, but the way people and even coaches do it:

- Is to be discouraged from!

Same thing, as with cars.

- Cars are safe.

- Yes, of course.

- As long as there is no driver inside!

- Afterwards, they become as safe as the driver.

- As soon as a person takes place behind the steering wheel, this paradigm becomes only as secure as the person himself (or herself)!

So, if you are no super-specialist with free weights, and are not eager to put your whole life and health to learn it.

- Just forget about it!

- It is too complicated for newbies, and sometimes even for specialists, if you could judge after all the injuries veterans inflicted on themselves.

CALISTHENICS

What remains is bodyweight training.

- You would say: - Could it also be dangerous?

- Of course, as any single thing in this world.

- But your bodyweight, you have always to deal with it, whether you like it or not.

- Isn't that so?

If you are overweight, or obese, this is the moment to take the right resolutions, and change your lifestyle and eating habits!

From the one hundred exercises known in Calisthenics and concerning the spine, I would propose you only 2:

- The simplest is the best!

You do not want to be encumbered by multiplicity.

What you are aiming at, is efficiency!

Those, which I found best for conditioning the spine, are:

1.   - Leg raises.
2.   - Push- ups.

As to how you should do them, you have plenty of

tutorials on Amazon.com or Kindle, or on Internet for free.

There are still a few things, which need consideration in this topic.

- Especially, because we do not have to deal with a normal spine, but with a spine with scoliosis.

Lessons from Weightlifting:

- What we learn from experience gathered in this community is:

1. - Exercising near to 100% Max (1RM) promotes joint problems.

Most professionals exercise with a repetition range of 3- 4, frequently 1- 2.

After a few years of this treatment, they all develop tendon or joint problems.

There are not many ways in which a joint adapts or tries to adapt to excessive strain.

Osteoarthritis is the result.

But radiological signs of osteoarthritis (arthrosis in Europe) are by no way the disease itself. They are only the result of it:

- I. e. an attempt of any given articulation to increase its portable surface, creating overhanging edges, called osteophytes. (Synonyms: bone spurs or parrot beaks).

Initial pathological process (physiopathology) has probably to do with joint capsule and its strength.

Training of any kind produces injury in muscle, on microscopical level, and hypertrophy is result of adaptation to resistance exercise.

This means that muscle fibers are destroyed in this process, as soon as ruptured, and new ones are implemented instead.

JOINT RESISTANCE

Concerning joints, it is probably the same process.

Ligament fibers are torn in strength training, are subsequently resorbed, and new ones, thicker and more resistant replace them.

Thus, observation of shoulder stabilization after habitual dislocation with Calisthenics. (See Vol. 1).

This happens only several months after beginning with strength training.
- Before cartilage rim could unit with articular cup (glenoid labrum).
- And before main ligaments could be rearranged (Middle gleno- humeral ligament rupture in antero-inferior dislocation of shoulder joint).

- Simply by tightening of all joint capsule fibers.

As we observed with this paradigm, disuse, i. e. abstaining from sports, leads to worsening of instability, while gentle resistance exercise leads to better joint stability.

Aerobics, on the contrary, instead of increasing stability, reduce it.

This means that there is a range of exercise in terms of %Max (1RM), that promotes tightening of articular capsule, while all training above and below this range, promotes an effect to the opposite, i. e. loosening of joint ligaments.

Aerobics means probably exercising below 10%Max (1RM).
- And implies presumptively lesser apposition of new ligament fibers.
- While Weightlifting means loads above 90%Max (1RM) and induces more ligament fibers destruction than apposition.

In both situations there is imbalance between positive and negative effect.

In the first, probably inhibition in reconstruction of new fibers, while in the second excess in destruction of such ones.

In researching literature, it seems that for upper extremities, safe range is about 70-80% Max (1RM), that corresponds to exercise in the 8- 10 repetition range.
- And for lower extremities, it is 50- 60% Max (1RM), that is in the 16- 20 repetition range.

Of course, this implies maximal loads much bigger

for legs than arms, as we are used to support all our weight on lower extremities all the time.

WEIGHTLIFTING

The result would be in Weightlifting, elaboration of safety rules, obliging practitioners to respect an eight repetitions range for training in clean and jerk and deadlift, and a sixteen repetitions range for squats.

For Calisthenics, it would mean to respect an 8- 10 repetitions range in any given step of increasing resistance, as for transition between two- and one-arm movements.

And of course, - a 16 repetitions range for the same topic concerning lower limbs.

The spine, as it belongs to mid- section, is somewhere in between, but as it is more supportive, than an actively moving structure, it lies probably somewhere nearer to upper limbs than to lower limbs.

So, if you ask in this respect:
- Which is safer?
- Calisthenics, or Weightlifting? T

The answer is without doubt, Weightlifting, as you

can titrate resistance by 1 lb. to the nearest of what you need.

CALISTHENICS

While with Calisthenics, you have more approximation, and between different levels of competency, you have frequently a jump of 30% in working load.

- That means you are training above your 90% Max (1RM).
- In practice trainers frequently propose to practitioners movements with only one repetition, which is near to 100%Max (1RM).

But, on the other side, you have fast adaptation with Calisthenics, at the expense of temporary instability (Vol.1- Shoulder dislocation).

While with Weightlifting you have no limit to the load you can put on your bar.

- As there is no limit to human greed.

In the first case adaptation with higher reps takes place before osteoarthritis installs, while in the second one, you end up with this disease after several years.

MILO

In the old Greek story of Milo of Kroton (sixth century BC), we all assume that the weight of his bull calf was corresponding to his 100% Max (1RM). Nothing is less sure than that!

In fact, probably, when his father would ask him how big his bull that day were, Milo would lift the animal 8 to 10 times, and then bring it to him.

So, the weight of that bull was near to Milo's 80% Max (1RM).

Otherwise, he would have suffered osteoarthritis after a few years, and would have been, by no way, able to participate in Olympic wrestling.

Historians tell us Milo of Kroton won six consecutive times the Games of Olympic wrestling between 540 and 516 BC.

These rules, if you want to accept them, for more safety in your sports practice, are correct, as long as we have to do with a normal joint.

As soon as we have a weak articulation, be it congenital, or acquired, you must implement different rules, and to refer to a different paradigm.

PARADIGM TMJ

The one I would like to propose to your attention, is the model of the temporomandibular joint.

Its articular surface does not exceed 0.5 cm2 (0.078 square inches).

This is so small, that even people who are simply chewing gum frequently, are bound to develop degenerative disease, within a few years, even a few months.

- Yes, many youngsters have osteoarthritis of their temporomandibular joint in early twenties.

If you consider what is the % Max (1RM) to which this joint has been subjected in this situation, it is no more than 20% Max (1RM).

- As this joint can sustain pressures of teeth loading, maximal for humans being in vicinity of 100- 200 kg (220lb- 440lb).

- This observation implies that for this joint, there is no safe range of strength training.

This paradigm also means, that for every joint surface, there is a maximal load to which it can be subjected safely.

RULES FOR SCOLIOSIS

So, if we return to our question:

- Which is safer, Calisthenics or Weightlifting?

You can give the answer, this time without hesitation.

- As this issue has not even been addressed as such by specialists in Weightlifting!

If now we return with this knowledge to our elaboration of rules for safety of lumbar spine in scoliosis:

- Rule N°1: Disuse is to be avoided, as it ends with loosening of joint capsule, same as aerobics.
- Rule N°2: Safe range of strength training depends on joint surface!
- Rule N°3: Safe Reps range would depend on degree of scoliosis. (This is corollary of Rule N°2).

If we try to envision such a system.
- But this is only a first attempt, which should be substantiated with results and experience

accordingly:

- For scoliosis of 5- 10° (Cobb's measurement):
- I would propose a repetitions range in Calisthenics between 16 and 20.
In this respect full range of motion is less of an issue, than repetition rate, and if you start with knee raises for instance, they should be incomplete.
- Or you can start at first with knee raises in recumbent position, as very first step of training.

- For scoliosis of 10- 20°: Repetitions range could be 25- 30.

- Extreme caution should be applied in more important grades of scoliosis, as functional articular surfaces in this condition are limited, like the temporomandibular joint!

- Corollary of these rules being:

- That above a particular grade of scoliosis any exercise could have deleterious results!
- Swimming could be proposed instead!

- Another situation, to be discussed:

- Is combination of a weak joint, as scoliosis for instance, and overweight, or obesity, at the same time.

- A weak joint would need as treatment tightening of its capsule, while obesity- dieting.

As diet means burning not only of body fat, but also of body proteins,

- All remodeling of tissue, involving last constituent, would be reduced.

Nothing is more deleterious to joint stability, than insufficient nutriment.

In this situation, you would have to choose between two options:

DIETING

- Either dieting or exercise!
- Of course, you could find a compromise in between, a bit of both!
- Corollary would be:
- Aiming at a higher repetitions range.

- Another situation, which should be addressed:

- How about an already present injury of spine.

- Let us consider the case of disc herniation.

- How does it occur?

Vertebrae are connected between themselves through two types of joints:

- 1. Intervertebral disc.
- 2. Posterior small articulations, called facets.

The first is a central gelatin ball (nucleus pulposus), contained through a tough capsule of ligament fibers (annulus fibrosus).

The second is a synovial joint.

DISC HERNIATION

A disc herniation is expansion of gelatin through a fissure in annulus fibrosus.

And travelling outside inter-vertebral space, compromising nerve roots, for instance.

This is a traumatic event.

It is always accompanied by pain. (As long as nervous system is safe).

As any single part of our bodies, also a disc herniation tends to heal.

It is a natural process, independent of surgery.

If gelatin of nucleus pulposus is in its normal location, it is nourished by repetitive motion of our bodies, which is repetition of higher and lower loading.

- As this occurs with every single step.

All nutrients are not transported by vessels till the center of the disc, as there are no such ones in this location, but by simple diffusion.

But as soon as gelatin arrives at another location,

surrounding vessels do not nourish it, but tend to reabsorb its water content.

The result is that it dries up.

During the same time, the fissure in annulus fibrosus, if not subjected to excessive load, tends to seal.

To promote and facilitate this normal process, specialists propose a bed rest of one to two weeks.

- Which is also the time needed for a scar in any tissue to consolidate.

If we consider purpose of exercise in this setting:

- We know from literature, that aerobics increase vascularity and perfusion of Musculo- skeletal system, while strength training promotes apposition of new ligament fibers.
- Hence place of physiotherapy in rehabilitation of modern neuro- surgery.

Engaging in Calisthenics program would come in third place.
- Aiming at strengthening of scar tissue in annulus fibrosus.
- And should be discussed only under supervision of neuro- surgeon and physiotherapist.

FATTY ACIDS

From another point of view the annulus fibrosus can be assimilated to a tendon.

Essential fatty acids, especially Omegas 3 and 6 are particularly important for health of such structures. Nutrition of modern population is largely deficient of those ones.

Omega 3 is contained in Linen oil, and Omega 6 in Safflower oil.

Those ones must be eaten raw in your salad or vegetables, because as soon you cook them essential fatty acids are lost. Cold pressed ones are the best.

I prescribe three teaspoons of each oil to my patients per day.

Colza oil is also very well balanced in those two essential fatty acids.

Sunflower oil contains them to an inconstant proportion.

WHIPLASH

Another topic is whiplash injury of cervical spine.

This is also a frequent traumatic event.

Consequences can be tremendous and dramatic, even with minor trauma.

Some can obviously be prevented by corresponding conditioning of this part of human skeleton.

This is common practice in the Boxing-, Wrestling- and MMA- communities.

As cervical spine is the smallest part of the whole spine, vertebrae in this location being one fourth of those of lumbar spine in size.

- Conditioning should be aimed at with a lot of caution.
- Highlight being on gentleness of all measures applied!

An exercise for the cervical spine that I like most is done lying down on the back and moving one's head from left to right and opposite, without any rotating motion.

People frequently neglect their health.

Professionals observe in patients with back problems relaxation of abdominal muscles (sign of disuse), and accentuation of lumbar lordosis.

This means that faulty working habits can induce even in normal spines a static flaw.

Many times, heavy duty jobs imply a working load of less than 10% Max (1RM) most of the time, with bouts above 90% Max (1RM).

The first promotes disuse, while the second is in the range of overload.

Conditioning, as outlined above, in vicinity of 80% Max (1RM), would preclude evolution towards osteoarthritis or disc herniation.

I hope this text would give you some incentive how to program a better future for yourself and your family!

WEBSITE

If you have any questions or comments, you can reach me at
www.thenopillshealthprospect.com